Essential DIY Cannabis Extracts and Concentrates:

Practical guide to original methods for marijuana extracts, oils and concentrates

By Anthony Green
Version 2.2
Published by HMPL Publishing at KDP
Get to know your publisher and his work at:
http://happyhealthygreen.life

A personal note from the writer

∽৩৫∾

In this practical guide, you'll find the most popular methods to prepare marijuana extractions. Everything is explained step by step, so you can get the most out of your bud. You'll learn how to make solvent-less concentrates such as dry sift hash, rosin, RSO and glycerine tincture; this book covers essential methods for cannabis extractions.

Read away, and cook up your medication to high-grade concentrates to get the best out of your product. The solvent-less methods provided are recommended to anyone that likes dabbing or smoking their medication.

Important note for patients that prefer to treat their condition with a tincture; we got you covered with the method for making this with vegetable glycerine! This guide also includes vital recipes to prepare the best coconut oil or cannabutter from the comfort of your kitchen.

If you're looking for the more traditional ways to make hash, such as Moroccan hash, the famous Afghan and Indian Charas, our book "Beyond Cannabis Extracts" is recommended.

In this extensive guide, you'll find all the traditional methods, as it goes deep into the subject of extraction.

This book only provides the essential methods for the most popular concentrates you want to make. You can find "Beyond Cannabis Extracts" here: http://bit.ly/CannaExtractsG

This is the no-nonsense approach to extractions and concentrates. I hope these methods fit your needs. If you have any questions during or after reading the book, please send me an email at hmpl.publishers@gmail.com

With kind regards,
Aaron Hammond

the publisher. The information herein is offered for informational purposes solely, and is universal as so. The presentation of the information is without contract or any type of guarantee assurance. The trademarks that are used are without any consent, and the publication of the trademark is without permission or backing by the trademark owner. All trademarks and brands within this book are for clarifying purposes only and are owned by the owners themselves, not affiliated with this document.

Disclaimer

The recipes provided in this report are for informational purposes only and are not intended to provide dietary advice. A medical practitioner should be consulted before making any changes in diet. Additionally, recipe cooking times may require adjustment depending on age and quality of appliances. Readers are strongly urged to take all precautions to ensure ingredients are of the highest quality.

The recipes and suggestions provided in this book are solely the opinion of the author. The author and publisher do not take any responsibility for any consequences that may result due to following the instructions provided in this book.

Table of Contents

oฆ฿o

Anthony Green

Bonus

⊰⊱

Welcome to HMPL Publishing! Let's start right away with an exclusive bonus made available only for our inner circle.

Get your free eBook **'The best DIY THC & CBD recipes to prepare at home'** here: http://eepurl.com/cxpVZf

Subscribing to our newsletter will get you the latest THC and CBD recipes, articles and some of our upcoming eBooks for absolutely free. To make that even better we'll update you with the most recent information about marijuana, medical breakthroughs, and the various applications of cannabis.

You can visit also http://happyhealthygreen.life

Or connect with us on Facebook; https://www.facebook.com/happyhealthygreen.life

The best methods of making hash, concentrates and extracts

∞૬ৈ৯৹

The methods of making traditional hash haven't changed much recently, but the modern methods that came along with legalization did. The quality and efficacy of extractions has improved a lot. With legalization on the rise, there is no need for cutting corners with low-grade plant material; so extremely potent and high-quality products are available to a much larger audience of consumers. Now this book gives you the opportunity to make the most out of your cannabis. To make your own high-quality medicinal products; these methods are the way go.

Whether you are a cultivator, extractor or a cannabis enthusiast; rosin and dry sift are definitely the most recommendable if you like to dab, smoke or vape your concentrate. Are you looking for a medicinal approach to cannabis? Try out the method for our glycerine-based tincture or medicate yourself with classic Rick Simpson Oil. If you prefer edibles, this book explains how to make the best cannabis infused butter and coconut oil. From the process of decarboxylation to measuring and dosing your edibles, this book provides everything you need to know! In the following chapters of this book, we talk about all these methods and explain in easy steps how to do it yourself.

***

CO2 cannabis extraction

❧❧

CO2 extraction is a method of extraction very similar to making Bubble hash with main and the only difference is that it takes using water out of the process by using dry ice.

Make sure you follow a few simple dry ice precautions while making your cold CO2 hash.

- ❖ Don't touch the dry ice without your gloves! You wouldn't want to get any freezer burns.

- ❖ Don't eat the dry ice.

- ❖ Don't place it in any airtight containers because you'll make them explode. Store it in a thick Styrofoam cooler to slow down the sublimation process.

- ❖ Make sure you work with dry ice in well-ventilated areas to avoid inhaling more carbon dioxide than you should.

- ❖ Safely dispose of any leftover dry ice by allowing it to warm up and transform back into harmless CO2 gas.

Supplies Needed:

- ❖ Good amount of great bud and top leaves
- ❖ Heat resistant gloves for handling the dry ice; you don't want to end up with freezer burns!
- ❖ Bubble Bag Kit in 220, 160, 120 and 70 microns
- ❖ 5gallon bucket
- ❖ A putty knife, paint scraper or just a laminated card to collect the kief hash
- ❖ A large clean mirror or piece of Plexiglas
- ❖ About 3 pounds of dry ice

Procedure:

1. Safety first, put your gloves on.
2. Grind your cannabis up and drop it in your 5-gallon bucket.
3. Cover it in dry ice.
4. Fit your 70 micron Bubble Bag over the opening of the bucket and shake the contents around for about 4 minutes to freeze the trichome resin off of the cannabis.
5. Lift the bucket up, turn it upside down over your clean mirror or Plexiglas and start shaking out as much cold powdery resin through the micro-mesh Bag as you can until you can't shake any-more out.

6. Use your scraper or card to smoothly scoop up the kief hash from your surface area into your mason jar.

7. Repeat the previous steps with the size-160 and 220 Bubble Hash Bags in order to collect three different grades of pure, solvent-free, homemade CO_2 hash which you can smoke, vape, dab or infuse into edibles!

***

Bubblehash and ice-o-lator

൦ക‍ന‍

Ice-o-lator or Bubble hash is an extremely potent kind of hash. Bubble hash thanks its potency to its special method of production involving extraction and sieving through ice-water. Precise THC content is always a bit of a guess unless you're able to have it tested, but bubble hash is one of the more potent forms of hash if you make it the right way.

Production:

The secret behind Bubble hash or ice-o-lator is in the method of making it. Using iced water and agitation in special Bubble Bags, you are able to separate the resin from the buds and icy water, and then collect the resin. The trichomes and resin found on buds are oily so that means that they simply do not mix with water which makes the process actually pretty simple.

Putting about 100 grams of good flower in iced water yields 10 grams of very high-quality hash. It simply requires putting your cannabis in water, agitating it with an egg beater or cake mixer for 15-20 minutes and then using a filtration system of micron filtered Bubble Bags. These are a set of bags that come with different micron sizes for the filter part at the bottom of each Bubble Bag.

Usually the bags range from micron filters of 220μ up to 70μ, with 70 microns being the finest filter able to sift through only the highest quality of crystals. This leaves you with a small amount of some very pure blonde resin. In the Bags with less than 70 microns you will have left over residue of flower but still very high-quality hash. We will explain this more thoroughly with dry sift hash as the method of extraction with Bubble Bags is fairly easy and the results are easily distinguished compared to dry sieve method.

Note: If you are using an electric mixing device, we recommend mixing in a separate bucket before pouring the mixture into your Bubble Bags and allowing it to settle.

The original Bubble Bag system which you can purchase online offers you eight layers of industrial grade micron filtration ranging from 220μ up to 70μ with 70 microns which will allow you to extract the perfect Bubble hash.

Supplies Needed:

- ❖ Good amount of great bud and top leaves
- ❖ Bubble Bag kit
- ❖ Bucket
- ❖ Hand mixer or a spoon big enough to stir up your bucket
- ❖ Tea towel

❖ Pressing screen

Procedure:

1. Line the bucket with your Bubble Bags, starting with the 25-micron Bag and ending with the 220-micron Bag.

2. Fill the bucket with enough cold water to cover the bottom of the Bubble Bags (about halfway full).

3. Add your dry or frozen plant trimmings.

4. Add enough ice to almost fill your bucket to the top.

5. Stir your mix for 15 to 20 minutes, adding ice if necessary to keep the water cold. A 50/50 mix of ice and water is ideal.

6. Pull out your Bubble Bags one by one, draining the leftover water in the Bag into the bucket.

7. As you pull each Bubble Bag from the bucket, turn it inside out after it is finished draining to collect your herbal extract.

8. Gently press the excess moisture out of your Bubble hash using your pressing screen and a dish towel.

***

Dry-sieve Hash

∽⊙⌒∾

Dry sift or kief is the result of mechanically removing the resin glands from the plant by sieving them with screens of different sizes, without any kind of solvent.

So let's see how you can make the purest possible dry sift separation. We will use an ancient technique used in many of the traditional ways of hash making in which we sieve and re-sieve the resin glands with screens of different micron sizes. We can use either sieving screens or bags; if you want to use Bubble Bags without the ice and water to make dry sift hash it will be harder as you will have to screen very tense.

Most modern sieving systems on the market developed to separate resin glands, as the popular Pollinator, have a 150-160 micron mesh to separate the resin glands; which pass through the mesh from the plant material. But, according to the theory that a lot of plant residue isn't as small as the pure resin, there are lots of particles that also pass through the screen which we don't want to be part of our hash. Therefore, you will need to use different screens with different micron sizes to continue separating the different qualities of particles of your raw resin. Normally, the best quality is where you find the higher proportion of trichome heads; larger than 70 microns and smaller than 120.

So, if you want the best possible quality results, filtering "downwards" with a 160-micron mesh is not enough. You should also perform a second sieve to get rid of those particles smaller than a certain size.

Supplies needed:

- ❖ Cured buds (amount depends on how much hash you want to make) 10 grams of good quality flower could potentially be 1 gram of quality sieve

- ❖ Screen sieves in the sizes: 160, 70 and 45 microns

- ❖ Oven plate (without anti stick! preferably glass, iron, ceramic) or a large dish to catch the material derived from the sieving process

- ❖ Grinder

Note: Always use a plate that's big enough to put the screens in as you don't want spill to any of your product. Beforehand; you should make sure that your flower won't stick to the surface of the oven plate; No anti-stick as you'll maybe have some kief that's a bit sticky but anti-stick ruins everything!

Procedure:

1. Put the screens (ranging from 45 on the bottom to 160 on top) in the oven plate or large dish.
2. Break up and grind your flower.

3. Put the flower straight from the grinder on to your 160-micron screen, and you can now either start sifting or grind more flower, repeating step 1 & 2.

4. Start sifting your ground up material by spreading it around the screen and applying a little bit of tension but keep it gentle.

5. Sift al the material as good as possible until there are no particles that could be sieved through the 160-micron screen left.

6. Take off the 160-micron screen and put it carefully aside in a safe place; not spilling the material as you could use it to make cannabutter afterwards.

7. Repeat the process of sifting with resulting resin on your 70-micron screen to get your 70 micron dry sieve hash; as you sieve this thoroughly as explained in step 4.

8. Take off your 70-micron screen and carefully put that aside as this is your first quality dry sieve hash.

9. Repeat the steps of sifting with the resulting kief left on the 45-micron screen.

10. After sifting through the 45 micron screen you will have your second quality hash left on this screen; preferably you'd want to mix the first and

the second quality hash to get the best taste experience and effects, as the 45 microns contains more of the terpenes providing taste compared to THC trichomes in the 70-micron hash.

11. The small amount left on your plate or dish can be scraped together with something like a credit card and will be your third and highest quality dry sieve hash.

Drying and storing cannabis resin

The best dry sift hash is usually collected from buds cured for about 4-6 months (always, depending on phenotypes, drying and storage methods, etc.). We can cure our buds before making hash or just dry our buds, make the hash and cure the resin. Obviously, it is much more convenient curing and storing resin than plants.

Cured resin is pressed more easily than non-cured glands, and is also more potent and flavorful. The ideal curing temperature is 37°C (98.6°F), and you should open your jars every 2-3 days to renew the air inside them.

You can also store resin pressed. If you choose to do so, the resin will keep its organoleptic features much better, since only the surface will oxidize while the inside will degrade much more slowly. It is also advisable if you're planning to smoke the resin on a metal screen; otherwise, the resin will pass through it if you don't use several screens together. The ideal shape for minimum oxidation is a ball or sphere. Never press a piece of hash if you think there's moisture on the resin; cure it properly and then press it. Otherwise, your hash can get spoiled in few days.

The best way to store our cured resin is inside an airtight container in the fridge, at low temperature and low humidity levels. If you want to store your hash for long periods with minimum degradation, and humidity; high temperatures and oxygen are the worst enemies. That's why the airtight container is definitely necessary.

For more hash making methods and a look at the traditional art of hash making be sure to check out our other book "Beyond Cannabis Extracts" at: http://bit.ly/CannaExtractsG, where we dive into the history and go in-depth about cannabis extractions and the how-to.

***

Cannabis oils, extracts and concentrates

∽⟨∘⟩∾

Cannabis concentrates and extracts have become ambiguous words in the cannabis industry recently. It could either refer to the wax you vaporize, the tincture used under your tongue, or the some of the many varieties of orally administered THC-free cannabis oil that has been changing attitudes toward cannabis everywhere in the past years. The future of cannabis is steering toward these potent concentrated forms, especially as the therapeutic potential of non-smoking methods is realized by the public.

Under the umbrella of cannabis concentrates falls any product procured through an extraction process. Extraction methods involving things like butane, alcohol, and CO_2 strip away the compounds from the cannabis plant, leaving behind a product with a very high concentration of cannabinoids packed in every drop. Some types of extracts have been tested as high as 90% in THC, while others are rich in non-psychoactive compounds like CBD and will deliver medical benefits to those who need CBD without inducing a high feeling.

We have talked a lot about traditional hash varieties and methods to produce some very high-quality hash yourself. Due to that high-quality of dry sift and Bubble hash you could definitely qualify them as extracts, especially if you would decide to purify them through a rosin press. That would turn them into a more glass, wax, or shatter like substance, able to purify your hash from most of the plant matter left in it; purifying your extraction. But when it comes to traditional hash I wouldn't put the name concentrate or extract on it because if you got a piece of Moroccan hash that has been tested around 20% THC, you're talking about 80% residual plant matter and other possible contents in your product which don't exactly classify as an extract in my book. Technically speaking it *is* extracted but the quality is too low. Back in the day; when we're talking the 90's and earlier, there was only hash, very good hash and hash oil, the last one being a true extract involving a solvent with a very high THC potency.

***

How to make cannabis oil

~~~

Before you start anything you should read this:

This is an urgent message from the writer to everyone considering using this method to extract their own cannabis oil. As you are working with alcohol as a solvent it is of the utmost importance that you are aware of your surroundings concerning open fires, stoves smoking and other situations that could mean potential harm and risk of catching fire!

This is an easy alcohol cannabis oil extraction method similar to the CBD extraction method in our book about CBD & Hemp-oil.

This process will yield you about two to four grams of extremely potent, medicinal-grade CBD oil that is suitable for ingestion. After you have a few practice runs, the entire process for small-batch edible oil production should take you about an hour, including around thirty minutes of cooking time. Grain alcohol is recommended for this process because it is the solvent least likely to leave you impurities or residue in the final product.

Supplies Needed:

❖ One ounce of dried, ground-up bud material or two to three ounces of ground, dried trim/shake

❖ One gallon of solvent (grain alcohol or other high-proof alcohol)

Never use rubbing alcohol as there are chemicals in there to make this unsuitable for human consumption and could potentially be very dangerous to your health!

❖ Medium-sized mixing bowl (glass is best, or ceramic)

❖ Strainer (cheesecloth/stainless steel kitchen sieve combo, or muslin bags, grain-steeping bags or even clean stockings/nylons)

❖ Catchment container

❖ Double boiler or a-bain Marie

❖ Kitchen utensils (large wooden spoon, silicone spatula, plastic syringe for dosage and dispensing of oil, funnel)

Your preparation area

❖ Heat Source: An electric stove in your kitchen would work well. It is more dangerous to use a gas stove (if that's what you have) since a gas stove uses an open flame - you must use extra caution with a gas stove as the flame can ignite your solvent - keep anything containing alcohol at least 3 feet away from the flame of a gas stove at all times. A portable electric burner or a large tea warmer also work well.

❖ Fire Extinguisher: you should already have one near your stove, but double-check to make sure it's there and not expired.

❖ Ventilation: your preparation space should be a large open area with excellent ventilation. Open any windows and have at least one fan moving the air around. Turn on the fan above the stove if it's available. Solvent fumes in the air can catch fire, so the best thing you can do to protect yourself during this process is to ensure there is good ventilation in your preparation space.

Procedure:

1. Get organized – Prepare your space, arrange your necessary equipment, find a level work area and make sure that it is clean and set up before starting

2. Place the ground-up cannabis material into the mixing bowl, making sure to leave some space for the solvent. Find a larger bowl before proceeding further, if necessary.

3. Completely cover the plant material with the alcohol, adding about an extra inch of solvent above the top level of plant matter.

4. Using the wooden spoon, agitate the cannabis material within the solvent for about three minutes. This enables the resin glands to dissolve into the solvent. Make sure that the plant matter is thoroughly saturated and has had a chance to expel its resin content.

5. Place a straining bag or sieve into the catchment container. Pour the dark green liquid from the mixing bowl into the bag or sieve; allow the liquid to be filtered completely and pour into the container. Gently massage the bag to squeeze out as much liquid as possible.

Note: At this point, you have the possibility to repeat the previous four steps in order to extract as much resin as possible into the solvent. This second wash should remove most of the remaining resin.

6. Pour the strained liquid into the double boiler or in the cooking pots (au-bain Marie; placing a smaller cooking pot in a bigger one, allowing to put water in the bottom pot to prevent the top pot from overheating or cooking too quickly). Fill the bottom of the double boiler or the bottom pot with an appropriate amount of water. If your alcohol resin solution does not all fit in the top of the double boiler or cooking pot, you can keep refilling the pot as you boil down the CBD oil, eventually processing all of the rinse liquid.

7. Place the double boiler over high heat until the

liquid begins to bubble, which is actually the alcohol evaporating. When it reaches the bubbling stage, turn off the burner – the residual heat contained in the water bath will continue heating the mixture, allowing the alcohol to evaporate.

8. If the mixture stops bubbling, it may be necessary to turn the heat back on, once or twice more. The evaporation step usually takes between fifteen and twenty-five minutes to complete.

Note: The mixture should continue bubbling throughout the evaporation process. As the alcohol level decreases, so will the amount of bubbles. It helps to occasionally mix the solution with the silicon spatula, scraping the sides of the pan as you mix.

***

Rick Simpson oil

❦

The story of Rick Simpson

After Rick Simpson suffered a serious head injury in 1997, he sought relief from his medical condition through the use of medicinal hemp oil. When Rick discovered that the oil with its high concentration of THC cured cancers and other illnesses, he tried to share it with as many people as he could, free of charge, and start curing and controlling literally hundreds of people's illnesses.

Now we have gone a long way in legalization and use of cannabis ever since 1997, but the method of Rick Simpson oil is still relevant today for people who like their medicine this way. So we will walk you through the steps of production. This method is similar to extracting cannabis oil with alcohol.

The method of making RSO (Rick Simpson Oil)

෯෯

Before you start anything you should read this: *This is an urgent message from the writer to everyone considering using this method to extract their own cannabis oil. As you are working with alcohol as a solvent it is of the utmost importance that you are aware of your surroundings concerning open fires, stoves smoking and other situations that could mean potential harm and risk of catching fire!*

Supplies Needed:

❖ One ounce of dried, ground-up bud material or two to three ounces of ground, dried trim/shake, Pick the strain that best fits your medical needs!

❖ One gallon of solvent (grain alcohol or other high-proof alcohol)

Never use rubbing alcohol as there are chemicals in there to make this unsuitable for human consumption and could potentially be very dangerous to your health!)

❖ Medium-sized mixing bowl (Glass is best, or ceramic)

❖ Strainer (A cheesecloth/stainless steel kitchen sieve combo, or muslin bags, grain-steeping bags or even clean stockings/nylons)

❖ Catchment container

❖ Double boiler or au-bain Marie

❖ Kitchen utensils (large wooden spoon, silicon spatula, plastic syringe for dosage and dispensing of oil, funnel)

Your preparation area

❖ Heat Source: An electric stove in your kitchen would work well. It is more dangerous to use a gas stove (if that's what you have) since a gas stove uses an open flame - you must use extra caution with a gas stove as the flame can ignite your solvent - keep anything containing alcohol at least 3 feet away from the flame of a gas stove at all times. A portable electric burner or a large tea warmer also work well.

❖ Fire Extinguisher: you should already have one near your stove, but double-check to make sure it's there and not expired

❖ Ventilation: your preparation space should be a large open area with excellent ventilation. Open any windows and have at least one fan moving the air around. Turn on the fan above the stove if it's available. Solvent fumes in the air can catch fire, so the best thing you can do to protect yourself during this process is to ensure there is good ventilation in your preparation space.

Procedure:

Note: Preparation is key! Make sure you have all the proper supplies ready BEFORE you get started. Make sure you have your double-boiler, your extra flat surface 3+ feet away from the stove, your cannabis (ground up), your bowl, and a bottle of your chosen solvent.

1. Place the ground-up cannabis material into the mixing bowl, making sure to leave some space for the solvent. Find a larger bowl before proceeding further, if necessary.

2. Completely cover the plant material with the alcohol, adding about an extra inch of solvent above the top level of plant matter.

3. Use the wooden spoon and start to agitate the Cannabis material within the solvent for about three minutes. This will enable the resin glands to dissolve into the alcohol. Make sure that the plant matter is thoroughly saturated and has had a chance to expel its resin content.

4. Place straining bag or sieve into the catchment container. Pour the dark green liquid from the mixing bowl into the bag or sieve; allow the liq-

uid to be filtered completely and pour into the container. Gently massage the bag in order to squeeze out as much liquid as possible.

Note: At this point, you have the possibility to repeat the previous four steps in order to extract as much resin as possible into the solvent. This second wash should remove most of the remaining resin.

5. Pour the strained liquid into the double boiler or in the cooking pots (au-bain Marie; placing a smaller cooking pot in a bigger one, allowing to put water in the bottom pot to prevent the top pot from overheating or cooking to quickly).

6. Fill the bottom of the double boiler or the bottom pot with an appropriate amount of water. If your alcohol-resin solution does not all fit in the top of the double boiler or cooking pot, you can keep refilling the pot as you boil down the CBD oil, eventually processing all of the rinse liquid.

7. Place the double boiler on high heat until the liquid begins to bubble, which is actually the alcohol evaporating. When it reaches the bubbling stage, turn off the burner – the residual heat contained in the water bath will continue heating the mixture, allowing the alcohol to evaporate.

8. If the mixture stops bubbling, it may be necessary to turn the heat back on, once or twice more. The evaporation step usually takes between fif-

teen and twenty-five minutes to complete.

Note: The mixture should continue bubbling throughout the evaporation process. As the alcohol level decreases, so will the amount of bubbles. It helps to occasionally mix the solution with the silicon spatula, scraping the sides of the pan as you stir.

If the liquid has stopped bubbling but is still runny, you may turn the heat back on low for a moment until it starts bubbling again. You should keep the heat just around the boiling point of alcohol.

Heat is not as important at this point. Even if this mixture cools down to room temperature which can be unlikely even in a cold room, the alcohol will all eventually evaporate away as long as you continue to stir.

9. You are done when the mixture stops boiling and takes on its desired consistency.

While the oil is relatively soft now, once it cools down it will become thicker, almost like putty. You should work quick and steady to place this mixture into a plastic syringe, which will make it easy to store and dispense your medicine. Remember, this is a lot of medicine, and the starting dose is half the size of a grain of rice.

10. Use a plastic syringe to draw up the oil - this will allow you to easily create individual portions in the future.

Quick Tip: Mix the warm cannabis oil with coconut or olive oil if you need to make less potent doses, or if you plan to use this topically on your skin.

For oral doses, you need to use plastic applicators or syringes with no needles. These are often used to dispense medicine for children and can be found at the drug store or grocery store.

Use the plunger of the syringe to slowly draw up the warm cannabis oil. The first few syringes will be easy to fill, but as you have less and less liquid remaining in the pan, it will become harder. That's totally normal.If there is some leftover cannabis oil which you cannot fit in a syringe, you can put the remaining oil in any sort of small closed container, and you will be able to use a toothpick to get tiny rice-sized pieces for individual portions after it cools.

The semi-runny oil will become much thicker after it cools - if the oil becomes too thick to push out of the syringe, simply run hot water over the syringe to soften the cannabis oil.

Store the cannabis oil in a cool, dark place such as a cabinet.

***

BHOs and the difference between shatter, glass, wax, and budder

৽৵৵

Shatter, wax, honeycomb, oil, crumble, sap, budder, pull-and-snap...these are some of the nicknames that cannabis extracts have earned through their rising popularity, prevalence, and diversification. If you've heard any of those words anywhere before, they were likely used to describe BHO also known as butane hash oil, CO2 oil, or similar hydrocarbon extracts. This list of descriptive subcategories might lead you to believe that we are talking about some stark differences between each one, but the division between glass-like shatter and crumbly wax is more superficial than you would expect.

So we are talking different varieties of the similar substances derived through different methods; the most common method that has been related to these varieties called wax, shatter, glass, and budder is BHO. Recent advancements in extraction technology have enabled the use of other solvents and over time a new method called rosin developed as a method of solventless extraction. The end product derived through those methods is a highly potent oil of varying consistencies most popularly used for vaporization and dabbing.

Shatter, glass, wax, and budder

Shatter, with its flawless amber glass transparency, has a reputation for being the purest and cleanest type of extract. But translucence isn't necessarily the way to tell signs of quality; the consistency and texture of oil come down to different factors entirely.

The reason this shatter comes out perfectly clear has to do with the molecules which, if left undisturbed, form a glass-like appearance. Heat, moisture, and high terpene contents can also affect the texture, turning oils into a runnier substance; hence the commonly used nickname "sap". Cannabis oils that have the consistency falling somewhere between glassy shatter and viscous sap are often referred to as "pull-and-snap".

The term wax refers to the softer, opaque oils in your concentrate that have lost their transparency after extraction. Unlike those of transparent oils, the molecules of cannabis wax have crystallized as a result of agitation. Light can't travel through those irregular molecular densities, and that refraction leaves us with solid, non-transparent oil.

Just as transparent oils span the spectrum between shatter and sap, wax can also take on different consistencies based on heat, moisture, and the texture of the oil. There are runny oils with more moisture that tend to form gooey waxes often called "budder," while the harder ones are likely to take on a soft, more brittle texture known as "crumble" or "honeycomb." The term "wax" can be used to describe all of these softer, solid textures.

How to make BHO

❧❧

First, here are some very important points you need to know about what you can expect.

Equipment: You'll need an extraction tube; these are available in different sizes according to the amount of material you want to use. Good quality butane preferably from the same shop as you're getting your extraction tube from as not every other commercially sold can of butane is usable for cannabis extraction due to other chemicals that might be in this butane.

Yield: from frosty some good trim, you should be able to get at least 10% yield. That means that if you start with 100grams of product, you should get at least 10grams of shatter. From good buds you can yield up to 22-23% yield, but usually, the results on flower are around 16-20% depending on the quality. With some less frosty strains, yields will be around 12-15%.

Material: If the material is bad, the end product will be bad. Plain and simple. You can't take brick weed and expect it to make good shatter. However, you are able to get a great BHO from simple frosty trim if it's dried and cured properly. The frostier the material that you're using, the more yield you will get from it.

Safety: What you might have heard about the dangers of BHO is true! There is a lot that could go wrong, with the worst thing possible: igniting the butane fumes. Let's say that you're producing some BHO on your back porch and it starts to get dark. You flip on the light switch. If there is any kind of spark, those highly flammable fumes will ignite. When you try to make BHO yourself, literally tape down the light switches so you or someone else can't accidentally turn on the light. Be sure to wear safety goggles. Butane will spatter out at some point, especially when you are still learning your equipment and finding the correct adapter from your butane can to the tube.

Supplies needed:

- ❖ 10 oz. can of butane per 1 oz. of marijuana
- ❖ Extraction tube
- ❖ Medium Pyrex dish
- ❖ Large Pyrex dish
- ❖ Electric heating pad
- ❖ Razor blade scraper
- ❖ Concentrate container
- ❖ A purging system (optional)

Procedure:

1. Extract the marijuana

First of all, fill your extraction tube with the strain you have chosen to process . Make sure to prevent any air pockets from forming and the material you are using is extremely dry. Fill the tube, pack it down, and then repeat until your tube is full and air-free.

For less plant material, use a smaller tube.

2. Fasten the screen (or a mesh coffee filter) to the bottom of the tube

Hold it over the medium Pyrex dish, then get your butane and put the nozzle right over the top hole in the tube. Allow the butane to flow into the tube, and then wait for up to a minute until the liquid begins to drip into the Pyrex dish. Use as many butane cans as necessary. Allow the drip to continue for several minutes. The liquid that you collect in your Pyrex dish should appear gold in color.

3. Once you have completed the extraction process

Now, you will need to evaporate the liquid so that the harmful butane can be removed. Get the large Pyrex dish and put the medium one inside of it. Then, put hot water in the outer, larger dish. This will cause the butane to begin to evaporate, which should take between fifteen and twenty minutes. Replace the hot water as needed to keep it hot. For your safety, be sure there is plenty of ventilation during this process.

4. Purge it

Purging is the process to complete the removal of the butane honey/hash oil. Using a purging system is the best way to do it, but many money-conscious people prefer to use an electric heating pad instead. Simply set it to high heat, and then place the medium Pyrex dish on it for an hour or more. Watch it carefully. This is finished once the oil stops bubbling.

Honey oil that has begun to become hazy or cloudy in appearance looks that way because of trapped butane. Purge it again to get rid of all the butane. One simple way of checking if there is any butane left in it is to touch it with a flame — if it catches, there is still butane that needs to be removed.

5. Store the oil

Use the razor blade scraper to get all of the oil out of the dish, and then put it all into a concentrate container. As long as it remains in an airtight container that remains dark and cool, BHO can last a long time. If improperly stored, you can expect the substance to become dry, tasteless, and less potent.

***

Rosin tech method for extraction

ⷎⷎ

Rosin Tech is by far the easiest method to extract your cannabis flower or any of your traditional hash and kief. It is a simple and affordable way to produce a quality product within seconds. This simple technique will separate the resin from the plant material by using heat and pressure. The resulting yields from this method are much similar to other extraction techniques, ranging between 10-15% with flower and much more with good quality hash like dry sift, bubble hash and kief.

Use the right tools

You can make rosin using most ordinary household hair straighteners or larger heat press systems such as t-shirt presses. Producing rosin press extracts requires a temperature between 240 and 330 degrees Fahrenheit on your ceramic plate. You will also need a heat source on both sides of the press. Any device that fits those criteria should work. You can purchase a hair straightener capable of making rosin for less than $20 for personal use. This is highly recommended for those planning on running up to a half ounce. Any more than that and you should look to invest in a heat press. This will run you several hundred dollars. The size of the ceramic plate on smaller devices matters less than you may think.

Small buds work the best if you're pressing cannabis flower

Think about it this way: using smaller nuggets to press creates more surface space overall. More surface space gives the resin a greater opportunity to reach parchment; the alternative being the oil will re-adhere to the starting material during the press. The good stuff collects in a ring around the starting material. Anything else is temporarily unobtainable unless you resort to running your chips over and over again. Doing this is not recommended. You will lose valuable terpenes each time you do. So take the time to break your starting material down to 1/2 inch to 1/3 inch bits. You may spend more time pressing, but the end result of your extraction will be worthwhile.

Listen while you press

This may sound strange, but the sizzle coming from your press is a great way to gauge when sublimation is occurring; sublimation is the point at which the oils change from a liquid to a gaseous state and then begins to look for something nonpolar to adhere to. Most of the time, this will only take about 5-7 second to hear this sizzle. After you hear it, let off the pressure a second or two later and remove the parchment from the heat source.

Temperature means everything!

Here is rough estimation that should help you with temperature.

Lower temperatures; 200's F, 90 -135 Celsius means more flavor, less yield, end material is more stable (shatter)

Higher temperatures; 300's F, 135 -185 Celsius means less flavor, more yield, end material is less stable and has a sap like consistency.

Do not go higher, this can be dangerous!

Use a screen to clean your extract

Get yourself a 25 Micron screen, because these are wonderful for processing kief and lower quality hash with. You can also use 90 micron tea filters to process flower with. Doing so will help keep all of the plant matter and particulates out of your end material. If you find that little pistils and other contaminants keep ending up in your flower rosin, use a dabber tool to remove them from the parchment before you collect. This should help!

Heat resistant gloves

Heat resistant gloves cost less than 10 dollars and will ensure that you don't burn yourself. Practice safety always!

The difference between strains

Your flavor and yield begin with your starting material. If the flower has poor resin, you will produce poor hash oil. Garbage material in means garbage results out. Remember this if you find you aren't achieving adequate yields. Also, certain strains are known for producing better resin than others. Do your research.

Before you collect it

After you press your starting material, let your parchment stabilize in the freezer for about 10 seconds. This helps with samples that lean towards the sappy side. Cooling it off will make it much easier to collect your extract onto your dabber tool.

Use a ball point dabber tool to collect

Ball point dabbers help you roll the tool over the paper. This ensures that you cover the most real estate. Sometimes, you might not be able to detect the rosin with your naked eye. However, rest assured that you are collecting material, even if you may not see it.

Supplies needed

- ❖ Any good amount of bud or quality hash
- ❖ Hair straightener with temperature control
- ❖ Non-stick parchment paper
- ❖ Collecting device such as a dabber tool, razor blade, etc.

❖ 25u micron screen

Procedure:

1. Prepare your processing material by breaking it down to 0.2 - 0.5-inch increments. Cut 10-20 pieces of parchment paper in 4" x 8" strips. Preheat the flat iron to 200F/93 Celsius – 340F/171 Celsius.

2. Take one of the small increments that you prepared and wrap them in the center of the 25u micron screen. Place the screen with the product on a piece of parchment paper and then fold the paper over, leaving the product in the center of your parchment paper. Place the parchment paper on the flat iron and apply pressure for 3-5 seconds directly on the product.

3. 3. Remove the pressure from the flat iron and take off the parchment paper, unfold the parchment paper. The starting product will be surrounded by the rosin, remove the product being careful to leave all of the rosin behind. Take your collecting device and scrape the parchment paper to collect the entire finished product.

***

Cannabis butter, oil and infusion methods for cooking with cannabis

⟪≈⟫

The most vital ingredient of making yourself some delicious edibles is the infusion of cannabis. Cannabinoids such as THC and CBD bind themselves to fatty acids so you got yourself a couple of options. The most common way is using butter as your medium of infusion. I, myself, prefer to use coconut oil, because it has a more efficient infusion rate compared to dairy butter.

For more cooking with cannabis and a look at the art of making edibles be sure to check out our other book "Cannabis Cookbook" at: http://amzn.to/2onxABM, where we dive into the subject and explain what you need to get the best out of cooking with marijuana.

Calculating edible potency

If I have 100g of top-shelf Blueberry, I would estimate the potency around approximately 18%, or about 180mg THCA per 1g of bud. So this means that 200mg of THCA x 100 is 18,000mg THCA.

The conversion from THCA to THC is 0.88 as I mentioned earlier. So this would mean that 18,000mg x 0.88 = 15,840 mg maximum THC available to be extracted.

Under the ideal conditions, you would get a 60% efficiency of extraction in dairy butter, so that means 15,840 mg x 0.6 = and you're looking at 9,504 mg maximum THC likely to be extracted.

In coconut oil you get 90% efficiency of extraction, which is why I choose to use that as my medium. That would mean that through the same process, 15,840 mg x 0,9 = 14,256 mg.

So with this knowledge, and if your targeted dosage is 200mg per brownie, then 14,256 / 200 = 71 brownies that contain around 200mg each. This is the maximum those brownies will have; they could potentially have a lot less depending on the infusion process and if it is done properly.

Decarboxylation and why is this absolutely necessary?

❦

Decarboxylation is turning your non-psychoactive THCA into THC for short. To understand this process, you have to start with the fact that all cannabinoids contained within the trichomes and resin of raw cannabis flowers have an extra carboxyl ring or group known as COOH attached to their chain. For example, THCA or tetrahydrocannabinol acid is synthesized within the trichome heads of freshly harvested cannabis flowers. In most regulated markets right now, cannabis distributed in dispensaries contains labels detailing the product's cannabinoid contents. THCA, in many cases, prevails as the highest cannabinoid present in items that have not been decarboxylated such as buds or hash and certain extractions.

THCA has a number of known health and medicinal benefits when consumed, including anti-inflammatory and neuroprotective qualities. But THCA is not psychoactive, and must be converted into THC through decarboxylation before any effects can be felt.

The two main reasons for decarboxylation to occur are heat and time. Drying and curing cannabis over time will cause a partial decarboxylation to occur. This is why some cannabis flowers also test for a presence of small amounts of THC along with THCA. Smoking and vaporizing will instantaneously decarboxylate cannabinoids due to the extremely high temperatures present, making them instantly available for absorption through inhalation.

While decarboxylated cannabinoids in vapor form can be easily absorbed in our lungs, edibles require these cannabinoids to be present in what we consume in order for our bodies to absorb them throughout digestion. Heating cannabinoids at a lower temperature over time allows us to decarboxylate the cannabinoids while preserving the material so you can infuse into your oil or butter to make edibles.

The THCA in cannabis begins to decarboxylate at approximately 104.4C or 220F after around 30-45 minutes of exposure. Full decarboxylation may require some more time to occur. I would choose to decarboxylate their cannabis at slightly lower temperatures for a much longer period of time in attempts to preserve terpenes. It makes up for some of the characteristics in taste of your flower, and also gives what you're eating a bit of a green taste.

Heat and time can also cause other forms of cannabinoid degradation to occur. For example, CBN (cannabinol) is formed through the degradation and oxidization of THC, a process that can occur alongside decarboxylation. CBN accounts for a much more sedative and less directly psychoactive experience.

In order to decarboxylate cannabis at home, all you need is some starting material, an oven set to 104-6C or 220-23F (depending on your location and oven model), some parchment paper, and a baking tray. Finely grind your cannabis until the material can be spread thin over the parchment and placed on your baking sheet. Allow the cannabis to bake for 45-60 minutes, or longer if would want that.

Always decarb your bud, kief, hash, or concentrate before you go for infusion in oil, butter or another solvent because even though part of that process happens though simmering your product, it has been shown that this comes nowhere close to the full potential of your material.

Clarified butter (Ghee)

৯৬৯৯

Clarified butter is used when you'll extraction cannabis in dairy butter. For those times when you want the flavor of butter, rather than oil, you'll want to use clarified butter which can stand being cooked longer, and to a higher temperature, than regular butter. This is very important as you don't want your butter to get burned and black with all your precious cannabis in there. The method of extraction takes at least an hour, and if you don't use clarified butter, you'll have to be very careful with your dairy butter! Coconut oil has a much higher burner point than butter altogether so that's another reason to pick coconut oil over dairy butter.

Clarifying butter removes the milk proteins and water, which are what causes the butter to burn if cooked for a long time. This ideal for infusing your cannabutter as you will need to simmer this for over an hour usually and regular butter easily burns over extended periods of simmering especially with flower in it.

Ingredients:

❖ Unsalted butter, cut into cubes

Tools:

- ❖ Heavy saucepan
- ❖ Spatula
- ❖ Fine steel strainer
- ❖ Cheesecloth
- ❖ Heat proof container

Procedure:

1. Heat the unsalted butter in a heavy-duty saucepan over very low heat, until it's melted. Let simmer gently until the foam rises to the top of the melted butter. The butter may splatter a bit, so be careful.

2. Once the butter stops spluttering, and no more foam seems to be rising to the surface, remove from heat and skim off the foam with a spoon.

3. Line a fine steel strainer with a few layers of cheesecloth or gauze, and set the strainer over a heatproof container.

4. Carefully pour the warm butter through the cheesecloth-lined strainer into the container, leaving behind any solids from the bottom of the pan.

Note: Clarified butter will keep for 3 to 6 months in the refrigerator. Some say you can leave it at room temperature if the conditions are optimal, but I keep mine under refrigeration. It can also be frozen for a longer length of time.

***

Double boiler method

When you put a pot on the stovetop, it gets hot especially the parts of the pot that make physical contact with the heating element, but for cannabis infusion this is not always the best way to go. Depending on your stove, things might get too hot too quickly; if your using normal dairy butter instead of clarified butter this can result in burning your butter in mere seconds. For clarified butter the burning point is much higher but you might get your oil too hot and lose THC in the process as this will vaporize. So the double boiler method gives the perfect opportunity to let your infusion simmer for hours around boiling point without getting too hot too fast and is easier to regulate just by adding cold water to the bottom pot.

A double boiler consists of a bowl or a smaller pot placed on top of a pan of simmering water. The bowl doesn't have to touch the water but creates a seal with the bottom pan to trap the steam produced by the simmering water. The trapped steam keeps the top bowl going at just about 100C (212F), the temperature at which water turns to steam and a far lower temperature than could be achieved by putting the bowl directly on that burner. Inside the top bowl, you can melt chocolate without worrying that it will stick and burn.

You can buy a double boiler, but it's easy to make one at home. All you need to make a double boiler is a mixing bowl (glass/Pyrex or metal) and a saucepan that the bowl will fit on top of. The two should fit tightly together; you don't want a gap between the bowl and the saucepan, nor do you want a bowl that sits precariously on a tiny saucepan. To use the double boiler, add water to the pan and bring it to a simmer, then place the bowl on top and fill it with whatever you intend to cook or melt.

Cannabutter

Ingredients:

- ❖ 1/2 oz. flowers
- ❖ 8 oz. clarified butter

Tools:

- ❖ Sheet pan
- ❖ Crockpot or double boiler method
- ❖ Fine steel strainer
- ❖ Cheesecloth

Procedure:

1. Preheat oven to 104°C or 220°F.
2. Grind your flowers down in a blender or food processor. Spread ground flowers evenly on bottom of a sheet pan and place in the middle of the oven.
3. Bake for an hour, stirring once halfway through. Make sure the flower stays evenly spread out.
4. Take the pan out of the oven and allow it to cool

down for 10 minutes.

5. Let the flowers sit for 10 to 15 minutes. Meanwhile, begin melting your butter over low heat.

   Since you have already decarboxylated, the butter only needs to be hot enough to extract cannabinoids. A slow simmer is good. Spoon the flower into the butter and stir. Extract using a crockpot or the double boiler method set on low for 6 hours and stir every hour or so to prevent burning.

6. Once your infusion is done, turn off heat and let the cannabutter cool down for at least 20 minutes.

7. Line a metal strainer with cheesecloth. Pour your butter through the cheesecloth and use a spoon to squeeze all the infused cannabutter out.

8. Now your cannabutter is ready to use in our recipes! Keep it in the fridge and use within two weeks or put it in the freezer and it will last you for about 4-6 months.

***

Cannabis infused coconut oil: The long method

❧❧

Ingredients:

Note: Make sure you have time for this as the process can take up 16-20 hours!

- ❖ Organic unrefined coconut oil
- ❖ 1-3 ounces of dried and decarbed cannabis
- ❖ Water

Tools:

- ❖ Crockpot
- ❖ Fine metal strainer
- ❖ Coffee grinder
- ❖ Cheesecloth
- ❖ Large container
- ❖ Thermometer

Pro tip: if you want to have less of a marijuana scent and taste to your final product leave your buds soaked in water overnight.

Procedure:

1. Grind the cannabis extremely fine. A coffee grinder works great, but make sure not to get it too powdery. This will make it harder to strain out in the final process.

2. In the crockpot, add the coconut oil and enough water to float the oil in the pot.

3. Set the heat on high and allow the oil to liquefy.

4. Slowly start stirring in the bud until the mixture is completely saturated. If needed, add more water.

5. Stick a thermometer in the pot with the lid closed on top, and monitor this closely it until it reaches close to 109C/250F. Turn the crockpot heat setting to low and stir.

Note: Oil continues to rise in temperature after being removed from heat, and takes longer to start cooling. So try to pre-emptive heat switch because this will help you keep a more accurate temperature.

6. Periodically stir the mixture and check that the temperature stays around 110 – 115C or 250 – 270F.

Note: An occasional flip from low heat to hot may be needed to regulate the temp.

7. The mixture needs to stay below 160C/320F to avoid burning off the active ingredient. The water

in the pot stops this from happening because it will evaporate first.

8. Periodically add water throughout the process to keep the cannabis submerged.

9. After 12 - 18 hours, turn off the crockpot and allow it to cool for a while.

10. Get the cheesecloth and double wrap it over your strainer. Place over a large container to catch the warm liquid.

11. Slowly pour the mixture into the cheesecloth and allow dripping. If it's not too hot, wrap the plant material and squeeze out the hot oil.

12. Continue until all the mixture has been squeezed out of the cheese cloth.

13. The remaining plant material can be saved to use for a topical compress. Although most of the medicinal properties lie within the oil still trapped in the spent bud.

14. Put the container of hot oil/water in the fridge overnight and allow the oil to rise to the top.

15. The water that was added during the process catches all the extra plant material and brown carcinogens from the mixture. This allows for a much cleaner tasting product.

16. Pop the hardened green coconut oil off the top of the water that sunk to the bottom, and discard of

the water.

17. You are now left with a green chunk of coconut oil that is ready to use for the recipe of your liking.

18. Store in the fridge until ready to use. Allow to warm before adding to recipes.

Pro Tip: Coconut oil is a good substitute for most baking and can replace butter in many recipes and some people like to add it to a hot beverage for an easy medication.

Cannabis infused coconut oil:
The short method

✤✤

Ingredients:

❖ Organic unrefined coconut oil

❖ 1 ounce or less of dried and decarbed cannabis

Tools:

❖ Spatula

❖ Double boilers or au-bain Marie

❖ Fine metal strainer

❖ Bowl or jar with a lid that fits with the metal strainer

❖ Jar with lid for storage

❖ Coffee grinder

❖ Cheesecloth

Procedure:

1. Grind up your bud but don't get as fine as possible, just broken up into smaller pieces will do perfectly.

Note: it is important that you are using an ounce or less of bud because the time of the cooking process would take a lot longer if you use more. If there is more product to be infused I would recommend using the long method.

2. Make sure it is decarbed before or after the grinding process by putting it on a dinner plate on a baking sheet in the oven for about an hour on 104C or 220F.

3. The ratio I like to use is 1:10 so 1 ounce of bud for ten ounces of butter, so put your double boiler on the stove, low heat, and add the coconut oil.

4. Stir until your oil is fully melted, stirring helps the coconut oil to melt a little faster.

5. Add your decarbed bud and stir again until your it's fully covered.

6. Let is simmer on low heat just keeping it around boiling point, 104C/220F should be perfect.

7. Stir occasionally every 5 to 10 minutes for about 1 to 2 hours.

Note: The oil will turn really dark and your bud will almost look burned with a slight smell of buttered popcorn and coconut oil to it, but don't worry that is part of the process.

8. After 1-2 hours turn off the heat and let it cool down, no need to rush this process.

9. After your product cooled down, you can either choose to take out the top pot from the double

boiler with your oil in it and put it in the freezer for two hours before straining it -- adding more potency to your infusion, or strain when it is cooled off and leave it in the fridge overnight.

10. Strain your oil by putting your steel strainer on a fitting bowl or jar, put the cheesecloth in your strainer, and slowly pour your oil and bud through the strainer.

11. If you used a jar with a lid you're finished and ready to store, keep it cool in the fridge or in the freezer, I personally prefer the latter.

12. Pour it from the bowl into your jar and store it.

Pro tip: Use the oil while it is cooled off but still liquid directly in your recipe; works perfectly with cake, cookies and brownies and makes the mixing process a lot easier! Make sure that it is cooled off as hot oil can burn or damage a plastic mixing bowl if you don't have a ceramic one.

***

Glycerin Tincture

✥✥✥

A glycerin tincture is cost effective and a safe way to medicate yourself with cannabis. It's also alcohol-free, which is amazing if you are sensitive to it. You can also customize this to fit your needs, just like cannabis coconut oil. You can use Sativa strains for daytime medication, high CBD strains for mood improvement, or Indica strains as medication for sleeping and pain relief.

The dosing for tinctures can be quite hard because you're most likely to be mixing up different strains and different materials to make it. This way you can't be entirely sure of the THC content of everything going in. This will take a bit of experimenting to figure out the best dose for you and your tolerance.

This tincture needs at least 60 days to finish but it takes very little effort during that time.

Supplies needed:

- ❖ Food-safe vegetable glycerin
- ❖ Decarboxylated sugar trim, kief, buds - even hash!
- ❖ Quart size mason jar

❖ Canning strainer stand + bag

❖ Glass bottles to store the tincture (something with a dropper will make it easy!)

Procedure:

1. **Prep work:** Start the procedure by decarbing your cannabis, Decarbing will keep you safe and make your tincture more potent. You have to ground your cannabis quite fine. You'll need to sanitize a large glass jar and any measuring or funneling equipment. *Note: this tincture will be taken orally it's very important to be careful about sanitation! You never want to make yourself or someone else sick.*

2. **Combine and let it sit:** Fill the jar at least 3/4 with your decarboxylated cannabis. Don't pack it in, just let it settle naturally. Once your cannabis product is in, pour vegetable glycerin over the top until the cannabis is entirely covered.

3. **What to do during the 60-day waiting period:** You don't need to do much, but it's a good idea to at least rotate the jar once a day.

4. **More decarbing:** Before you strain your tincture; there is one last thing you can do: decarboxylate. It is best to pour the tincture into a small crockpot or pan cover this with a lid because you don't want to have any cannabinoids escaping

your tincture and put it in well covered in the oven at 104C/220F for about an hour.

5. **Straining:** Using a canning strainer stand and bag is one of the simplest ways to do this. Just set up your stand and attach the straining bag firmly with a couple knots - it will be weighed down by the tincture and you don't want it to fall into the bowl below. Pour the entire contents of the jar into the strainer bag and let it sit overnight if you can. It will take a long time to drip through! Either wrap around the bottom vessel with plastic wrap to keep it free from debris or place it in a clean, cool place where it won't get knocked over.

6. **Storage and applications:** Vegetable glycerin has a shelf life of 14-24 months, keep it cooled in the fridge.

To use, simply take a bit orally. You can take it straight OR add it to tea, coffee, or whatever else you're drinking. The vegetable glycerin gives it a very sweet taste. This works well in drinks and smoothies.

***

Bonus reminder

⊰⊱

Welcome to HMPL Publishing! Let's start right away with an exclusive bonus made available only for our inner circle.

Get your free eBook **'The best DIY THC & CBD recipes to prepare at home'** here: http://eepurl.com/cxpVZf

Subscribing to our newsletter will get you the latest THC and CBD recipes, articles and some of our upcoming eBooks for absolutely free. To make that even better we'll update you with the most recent information about marijuana, medical breakthroughs, and the various applications of cannabis.

You can visit also http://happyhealthygreen.life

Or connect with us on Facebook; https://www.facebook.com/happyhealthygreen.life

www.ingramcontent.com/pod-product-compliance
Lightning Source LLC
Chambersburg PA
CBHW061050220326
41597CB00018BA/2727